The Pegan Diet Cookbook for Beginners

Enjoy this Complete Collection of Pegan Diet Recipes

Elena Rose

Table of Contents

Full-Flavored Vanilla Ice Cream

Preparation Time: 15minutes

Cooking time: 0minutes

Servings: 4

Ingredients

- 1 1/2 cups canned coconut milk

- 1 cup coconut whipping cream

- 1 frozen banana cut into chunks

- 1 cup vanilla sugar

- 3 Tbsp. apple sauce

- 2 tsp. pure vanilla extract

- 1 tsp. Xanthan gum or agar-agar thickening agent

Directions:

1. Merge all ingredients; process until all ingredients combined well.

2. Place the ice cream mixture in a freezer-safe container with a lid over.

3. Freeze for at least 4 hours.

4. Remove frozen mixture to a bowl and beat with a mixer to break up the ice crystals.

5. Repeat this process 3 to 4 times.

6. Let the ice cream at room temperature for 15 minutes before serving.

Nutrition:

Calories 126.89

Calories from Fat 134.39 |

Total Fat 15.6g

Saturated Fat 19.84g

Cholesterol 0mg

Sodium 28.19mg

Potassium 22

Total Carbohydrates 10g

Fiber 2.16g

Sugar 7.7g

Protein 5g

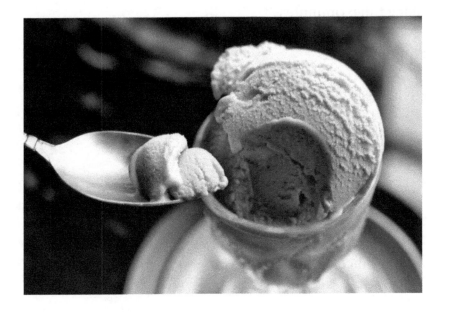

Irresistible Peanut Cookies

Preparation Time: 20minutes

Cooking time: 0minutes

Servings: 6

Ingredients

- 4 Tbsp. all-purpose flour

- 1 tsp. baking soda

- Pinch of salt

- 1/3 cup granulated sugar

- 1/3 cup peanut butter softened

- 3 Tbsp. applesauce

- 1/2 tsp. pure vanilla extract

Directions:

1. Preheat oven to 350 F.

2. Combine the flour, baking soda, salt, and sugar in a mixing bowl; stir.

3. Merge all remaining ingredients

4. Roll dough into cookie balls/patties.

5. Arrange your cookies onto greased (with oil or cooking spray) baking sheet.

6. Let cool before removing from tray.

7. Take out cookies from the tray and let cool completely.

8. Place your peanut butter cookies in an airtight container, and keep refrigerated up to 10 days.

Nutrition: Calories 116.89
Calories from Fat 114.39
Total Fat 18.6g

Saturated Fat 20.84g

Cholesterol 0mg

Sodium 12.19mg

Potassium 22

Total Carbohydrates 10g

Fiber 2.16g

Sugar 7.7g

Protein 5g

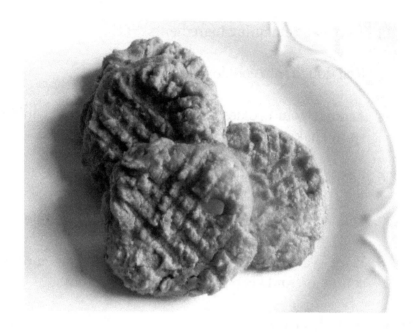

Murky Almond Cookies

Preparation Time: 10minutes

Cooking time: 15minutes

Servings: 6

Ingredients

- 4 Tbsp. cocoa powder

- 2 cups almond flour

- 1/4 tsp. salt

- 1/2 tsp. baking soda

- 5 Tbsp. coconut oil melted

- 2 Tbsp. almond milk

- 1 1/2 tsp. almond extract

- 1 tsp. vanilla extract

- 4 Tbsp. corn syrup or honey

Directions:

1. Preheat oven to 340 F degrees.

2. Grease a large baking sheet; set aside.

3. Merge the cocoa powder, almond flour, salt, and baking soda.

4. Merge the melted coconut oil, almond milk; almond and vanilla extract, and corn syrup or honey.

5. Merge the almond flour mixture with the almond milk mixture and stir well.

6. Roll tablespoons of the dough into balls, and arrange onto a prepared baking sheet.

7. Bake for 12 to 15 minutes.

8. Remove from the oven and transfer onto a plate lined with a paper towel.

9. Allow cookies to cool down completely and store in an airtight container at room temperature for about four days.

Nutrition:

Calories 16.89

Calories from Fat 19.39 |

Total Fat 18.6g

Saturated Fat 20.84g
Potassium 22

Total Carbohydrates 10g

Fiber 2.16g

Sugar 7.7g

Protein 5g

Orange Semolina Halva

Preparation Time: 10minutes

Cooking time: 25minutes

Servings: 6

Ingredients

- 6 cups fresh orange juice

- Zest from 3 oranges

- 3 cups brown sugar

- 1 1/4 cup semolina flour

- 1 Tbsp. almond butter (plain, unsalted)

- 4 Tbsp. ground almond

- 1/4 tsp. cinnamon

Directions:

1. Heat the orange juice, orange zest with brown sugar in a pot.

2. Let the sugar dissolved.

3. Add the semolina flour and cook over low heat for 15 minutes; stir occasionally.

4. Add almond butter, ground almonds, and cinnamon, and stir well.

5. Cook, frequently stirring, for further 5 minutes.

6. Transfer the halva mixture into a mold, let it cool and refrigerate for at least 4 hours.

7. Keep refrigerated in a sealed container for one week.

Nutrition:

Calories 16.89

Calories from Fat 19.39 |

Total Fat 18.6g

Saturated Fat 20.84g

Cholesterol 0mg

Sodium 12.19mg

Potassium 22

Total Carbohydrates 10g

Fiber 2.16g

Sugar 7.7g

Protein 5g

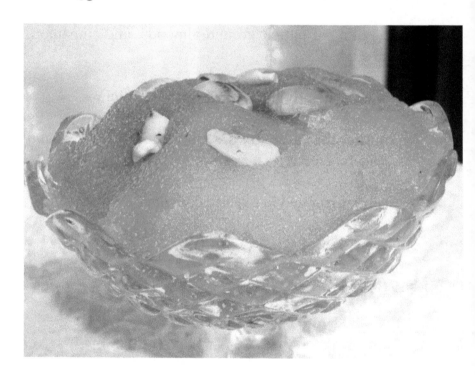

Seasoned Cinnamon Mango Popsicles

Preparation Time: 15minutes

Cooking time: 0minutes
Servings: 6

Ingredients

- 1 1/2 cups of mango pulp

- 1 mango cut in cubes

- 1 cup brown sugar (packed)

- 2 Tbsp. lemon juice freshly squeezed

- 1 tsp. cinnamon

- 1 pinch of salt

Directions:

1. Add all ingredients into your blender.

2. Blend until brown sugar dissolved.

3. Pour the mango mixture evenly in Popsicle molds or cups.

4. Insert sticks into each mold.

5. Place molds in a freezer, and freeze for at least 5 to6 hours.

6. Before serving, un-mold easy your popsicles placing molds under lukewarm water.

Nutrition: Calories 16.89 Calories from Fat 19.39 | Total Fat 18.6g Saturated Fat 20.84g Cholesterol 0mg Sodium 12.19mg Potassium 22

Total Carbohydrates 10g Fiber 2.16g
Sugar 7.7g Protein 5g

Strawberry Molasses Ice Cream

Preparation Time: 20minutes

Cooking time: 0minutes

Servings: 9

Ingredients

- 1 lb. strawberries

- 3/4 cup coconut palm sugar

- 1 cup coconut cream

- 1 Tbsp. molasses

- 1 tsp. balsamic vinegar

- 1/2 tsp. agar-agar

- 1/2 tsp. pure strawberry extract

Directions:
1. Add strawberries, date sugar, and the balsamic vinegar in a blender; blend until completely combined.

2. Place the mixture in the refrigerator for one hour.

3. In a mixing bowl, beat the coconut cream with an electric mixer to make a thick mixture.

4. Add molasses, balsamic vinegar, agar-agar, and beat for further one minute or until combined well.

5. Add the strawberry mixture and beat again for 2 minutes.

6. Pour ice cream mix into an ice cream maker, turn on the machine, and churn according to manufacturer's directions.

7. Keep frozen in a freezer-safe container (with plastic film and lid over).

Nutrition:

Calories 16.89

Calories from Fat 19.39 |

Total Fat 18.6g

Saturated Fat 20.84g

Cholesterol 0mg

Sodium 12.19mg

Potassium 22

Total Carbohydrates 10g

Fiber 2.16g

Sugar 7.7g

Protein 5g

Strawberry-Mint Sorbet

Preparation Time: 15minutes

Cooking time: 0minutes

Servings: 6

Ingredients

- 1 cup of granulated sugar

- 1 cup of orange juice

- 1 lb. frozen strawberries

- 1 tsp. pure peppermint extract

Directions:

1. Add sugar and orange juice in a saucepan.

2. Stir over high heat and boil for 5 minutes or until sugar dissolves.

3. Remove from the heat and let it cool down.

4. Add strawberries into a blender, and blend until smooth.

5. Pour syrup into strawberries, add peppermint extract and stir until all ingredients combined well.

6. Transfer mixture to a storage container, cover tightly, and freeze until ready to serve.

Nutrition:

Calories 16.89

Calories from Fat 1.39 |

Total Fat 12.6g
Saturated Fat 2.84g

Cholesterol 0mg

Sodium 1.19mg

Potassium 22

Total Carbohydrates 10g

Fiber 2.16g

Sugar 33g

Protein 5g

Vegan Choco - Hazelnut Spread

Preparation Time: 15minutes

Cooking time: 0minutes

Servings: 5

Ingredients

- 1 cup hazelnuts soaked

- 4 Tbsp. dry cacao powder

- 4 Tbsp. Maple syrup

- 1 tsp. pure vanilla extract

- 1/4 tsp. kosher salt

- 4 Tbsp. almond milk

Directions:

1. Soak hazelnuts with water overnight.

2. Add soaked hazelnuts along with all remaining ingredients in a food processor.

3. Process for about 10 minutes or until a cream gets the desired consistency.

4. Keep the spread in a sealed container refrigerated up to 2 weeks.

Nutrition:

Calories 16.89

Calories from Fat 4.39 |

Total Fat 6.6g

Saturated Fat 3.84g

Cholesterol 0mg

Sodium 5.19mg

Potassium 22

Total Carbohydrates 10g

Fiber 2.16g

Sugar 43g

Protein 5g

Vegan Exotic Chocolate Mousse

Preparation Time: 10minutes

Cooking time: 0minutes

Servings: 4
Ingredients:

- 2 frozen bananas chunks

- 2 avocados

- 1/3 cup of dates

- 4 Tbsp. cocoa powder

- 1/2 cup of fresh orange juice

- Zest, from 1 orange

Directions:

1. Add bananas, avocado, and dates in a food processor.

2. Process for about 2 to 3 minutes until combined well.

3. Add cocoa powder, orange juice, and orange zest; process for further one minute.

4. Place cream in a glass jar or container and keep refrigerated up to one week.

5. Nutrition: Facts

Nutrition:

Calories 16.89

Calories from Fat 4.39 |

Total Fat 5.6g

Saturated Fat 2.84g

Cholesterol 0mg

Sodium 7.19mg

Potassium 32

Total Carbohydrates 10g

Fiber 2.16g

Sugar 43g

Protein 5g

Vegan Lemon Pudding

Preparation Time: 20minutes

Cooking time: 0minutes

Servings: 6

Ingredients

- 2 cups almond milk

- 3 Tbsp. of corn flour

- 2 Tbsp. of all-purpose flour

- 1 cup of sugar granulated

- 1/4 cup almond butter (plain, unsalted)

- 1 tsp. lemon zest

- 1/3 cup fresh lemon juice

Directions:

1. Add the almond milk with corn flour, flour, and sugar in a saucepan.

2. Cook, frequently stirring, until sugar dissolved, and all ingredients combine well (for about 5 to 7 minutes over medium heat).

3. Add the almond butter, lemon zest, and lemon juice.

4. Cook, frequently stirring, for further 5 to 6 minutes.

5. Remove the lemon pudding from the heat and allow it to cool completely.

6. Pour into the sealed container and keep refrigerated up to one week.

Nutrition: Calories 16.89 Calories from Fat 7.39 | Total Fat 3.6g Saturated Fat 1.84g Cholesterol 0mg Sodium 7.19mg Potassium432

Total Carbohydrates 20g Fiber 1.16g
Sugar 24g Protein 5g

Vitamin Blast Tropical Sherbet

Preparation Time: 15minutes

Cooking time: 0minutes

Servings: 8

Ingredients

- 4 cups mangos pitted and cut into 1/2-inch dice

- 1 papaya cut into 1/2-inch dice

- 1/4 cup granulated sugar or honey (optional)

- 1 cup pineapple juice canned

- 1/4 cup coconut milk

- 2 Tbsp. coconut cream

- 1 fresh lime juice

Directions:
1. Add all ingredients into your food processor; process until all ingredients smooth and combine well.

2. Put the mixture to a bowl, and cover

3. Remove the sherbet mixture from the fridge, stir well, and pour in a freezer-safe container (with plastic film and lid over).

4. Keep frozen.

5. Let the sherbet at room temperature for 15 minutes before serving.

Nutrition:

Calories 16.89

Calories from Fat 9.39 |

Total Fat 2.6g
Saturated Fat 3.84g

Cholesterol 0mg

Sodium 7.15mg

Potassium132

Total Carbohydrates 15g

Fiber 1.16g

Sugar 24g

Protein 5g

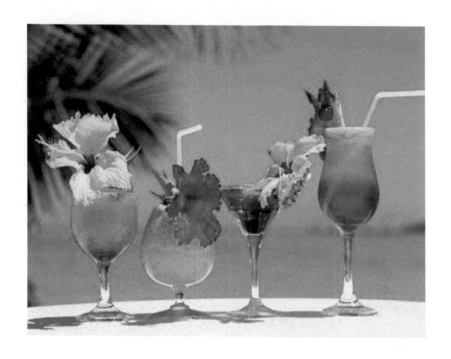

Walnut Vanilla Popsicles

Preparation Time: 15minutes

Cooking time: 0minutes

Servings: 7

Ingredients

- 1 1/2 cup finely sliced walnuts

- 4 cups of almond milk

- 4 Tbsp. brown sugar (packed)

- 1 scoop protein powder (pea or soy)

- 2 tsp. pure vanilla extract

Directions:

1. Add all ingredients in your high-speed blender and blend until smooth and combined well.

2. Pour the mixture in Popsicle molds and insert the wooden stick into the middle of each mold.

3. Freeze until your ice popsicles are completely frozen.

4. Serve and enjoy!

Nutrition:

Calories 16.89

Calories from Fat 9.39 |

Total Fat 2.6g

Saturated Fat 3.84g

Cholesterol 0mg

Sodium 7.15mg

Potassium122

Total Carbohydrates 15g

Fiber 1.16g

Sugar 34g

Protein 5g

Lentil-Quinoa Chili

Preparation time: 15minutes

Cooking time: 30minutes

Servings: 4

Ingredients:

- 1/2 cup dry green lentils

- 1 can black beans

- 1/3 cup uncooked quinoa, rinsed

- 1 small yellow onion, diced

- 2 medium carrots, diced

- 2 teaspoons ground cumin

- 2 teaspoons chili powder

- 1.1/2 teaspoons minced garlic (3 cloves)

- 1 teaspoon dried oregano

- 3 vegetable bouillon cubes

- 1 bay leaf

- 4 cups water

- Pinch salt

Directions:

1. Place the lentils, black beans, quinoa, onion, carrots, cumin, chili powder, garlic, oregano, bouillon cubes, bay leaf, and water in a slow cooker; mix well.

2. Cook on low heat.

3. Remove the bay leaf, season with salt, and serve.

Nutrition:

Calories: 617

Total fat: 2g

Protein: 72g

Sodium: 346

Fat: 16g

Eggplant Curry

Preparation time: 15minutes

Cooking time: 35minutes

Servings: 5

Ingredients:

- 5 cups chopped eggplant

- 4 cups chopped zucchini

- 2 cups stemmed and chopped kale

- 1 (15-ounce) can full-fat coconut milk

- 1 (14.5-ounce) can diced tomatoes, drained

- 1 (6-ounce) can tomato paste

- 1 medium yellow onion, chopped

- 2 teaspoons minced garlic (4 cloves)

- 1 tablespoon curry powder

- 1 tablespoon gram masala

- 1/4 teaspoon cayenne pepper

- 1/4 teaspoon ground cumin

- 1 teaspoon salt

- Cooked rice, for serving

Directions:

1. Combine the eggplant, zucchini, kale, coconut milk, diced tomatoes, tomato paste, onion, garlic, curry powder, gram masala, cayenne pepper, cumin, and salt in a slow cooker; mix well.

2. Cook on low heat.

Nutrition:

Calories: 417

Total fat: 2g

Protein: 72g

Sodium: 346

Fat: 19g

Meaty Chili

Preparation time: 15minutes

Cooking time: 40minutes

Servings: 5

Ingredients:

- 1 tablespoon olive oil

- 2 packages of faux-ground-beef veggie crumble (such as Beyond Meat)

- 1 large red onion, chopped

- 1 large jalapeño pepper, seeded and chopped

- 2 1/2 teaspoons minced garlic

- 1 can diced tomatoes
- 1 can kidney beans

- 1 can black beans

- 1/2 cup frozen corn

- 1/4 cup chili powder

- 2 tablespoons ground cumin

- 1 teaspoon smoked paprika

- 1 vegetable bouillon cube

- 1.1/2 cups water

Directions:

1. Heat the olive oil in a sauté pan over medium-high heat. Add the veggie crumbles, onion, jalapeño, and garlic, and cook for 3 to 4 minutes, stirring occasionally.

2. Combine the veggie-crumble mixture, diced tomatoes, kidney beans, black beans, frozen corn, chili powder, cumin, smoked paprika, bouillon cube, and water in a slow cooker; mix well.

3. Cook on low heat.

Nutrition:

Calories: 547

Total fat: 8g

Protein: 62g

Sodium: 346

Fat: 19g

Sweet Potato Bisque

Preparation time: 15minutes

Cooking time: 45minutes

Servings: 4

Ingredients:

- 2 sweet potatoes, peeled and sliced

- 2 cups frozen butternut squash

- 2 (14.5-ounce) cans full-fat coconut milk

- 1 medium yellow onion, sliced

- 1 teaspoon minced garlic (2 cloves)

- 1 tablespoon dried basil

- 1 tablespoon chili powder

- 1 tablespoon ground cumin

- 1/2 cup water

- Pinch salt

- Freshly ground black pepper

Directions:

1. Combine the sweet potatoes, butternut squash, coconut milk, onion, garlic, dried basil, chili powder, cumin, and water in a slow cooker; mix well.

2. Cook on low heat.

3. Blend the soup until it's nice and creamy.

   Season with salt and pepper.

Nutrition: Calories: 447 Total fat: 8g Protein: 72g Sodium: 346 Fat: 19g

Chickpea Medley

Preparation time: 5minutes

Cooking time: 15minutes

Servings: 4

Ingredients:

- 2 tablespoons tahini

- 2 tablespoons coconut amines

- 1 (15-ounce) can chickpeas or 1.1/2 cups cooked chickpeas, rinsed and drained

- 1 cup finely chopped lightly packed spinach

- Carrot, peeled and grated

Directions:

1. Merge together the tahini and coconut amines in a bowl.

2. Add the chickpeas, spinach, and carrot to the bowl. Stir well and serve at room temperature.

3. *Simple Swap*: Coconut amines are almost like a sweeter, mellower version of soy sauce. However, if you want to use regular soy sauce or tamari, just use 11/2 tablespoons and add a dash of maple syrup or agave nectar to balance out the saltiness.

Nutrition:

Calories: 437

Total fat: 8g

Protein: 92g

Sodium: 246

Fat: 19g

Pasta with Lemon and Artichokes

Preparation time: 10minutes

Cooking time: 20minutes

Servings: 4

Ingredients:

- 16 ounces linguine or angel hair pasta

- 1/4 cup extra-virgin olive oil

- 8 garlic cloves, finely minced or pressed

- 2 (15-ounce) jars water-packed artichoke hearts, drained and quartered

- 2 tablespoons freshly squeezed lemon juice

-
  1/4 cup thinly sliced fresh basil
- 1 teaspoon sea salt

- Freshly ground black pepper

Directions:

1. Use a large pot of water to a boil over high heat and cook the pasta until al dente according to the directions on the package.

2. While the pasta is cooking, heat the oil in a skillet over medium heat and cook the garlic, stirring often, for 1 to 2 minutes until it just begins to brown. Toss the garlic with the artichokes in a large bowl.

3. When the pasta is done, drain it and add it to the artichoke mixture, then add the lemon juice, basil, salt, and pepper. Gently stir and serve.

Nutrition:

Calories: 237

Total fat: 7g

Protein: 52g

Sodium: 346

Fat: 19g

Roasted Pine Nut Orzo

Preparation time: 10minutes

Cooking time: 15minutes

Servings: 3

Ingredients:

- 16 ounces orzo

- 1 cup diced roasted red peppers

- 1/4 cup pitted, chopped Klamath olives

- 4 garlic cloves, minced or pressed

- 3 tablespoons olive oil

- 1.1/2 tablespoons squeezed lemon juice

- 2 teaspoons balsamic vinegar

- 1 teaspoon sea salt

- 1/4 cup pine nuts

- 1/4 cup packed thinly sliced or torn fresh basil

Directions:

1. Use a large pot of water to a boil over medium-high heat and add the orzo. Cook, stirring often, for 10 minutes, or until the orzo has a chewy and firm texture. Drain well.

2. While the orzo is cooking, in a large bowl, combine the peppers, olives, garlic, olive oil, lemon juice, vinegar, and salt. Stir well.

3. In a dry skillet toasts the pine nuts over medium-low heat until aromatic and lightly browned, shaking the pan often so that they cook evenly

4. Upon reaching the desired texture and add it to the sauce mixture within a minute or so, to avoid clumping.

Nutrition:

Calories: 537

Total fat: 7g
Protein: 72g

Sodium: 246

Fat: 19g

Eggplant and Peppers Soup

Preparation time: 10 minutes

Cooking time: 40 minutes

Servings: 4

Ingredients:

- 2 red bell peppers, chopped

- 3 scallions, chopped

- 3 garlic cloves, minced

- 2 tablespoon olive oil

- Salt and black pepper to the taste

- 5 cups vegetable stock

- 1 bay leaf

- 1/2 cup coconut cream

- 1-pound eggplants, roughly cubed

- 2 tablespoons basil, chopped

Directions:

1. Heat up a pot with the oil over medium heat; add the scallions and the garlic and sauté for 5 minutes.

2. Add the peppers and the eggplants and sauté for 5 minutes more.

3. Add the remaining ingredients, toss, bring to a simmer, cook for 30 minutes, ladle into bowls and serve for lunch.
4. Nutrition:

Calories: 119

Total fat: 8g

Saturated fat: 6g

Sodium: 116mg

Carbs: 17g

Fiber: 9g

Protein: 6g

Cauliflower and Artichokes Soup

Preparation time: 10 minutes

Cooking time: 25 minutes

Servings: 4

Ingredients:

- 1 pound cauliflower florets

- 1 cup canned artichoke hearts

- 2 scallions, chopped

- 2 tablespoons olive oil

- 2 garlic cloves, minced

- 6 cups vegetable stock

- Salt and black pepper to the taste

- 2/3 cup coconut cream

- 2 tablespoons cilantro, chopped

Directions:

1. Heat up a pot with the oil over medium heat; add the scallions and the garlic and sauté for 5 minutes.

2. Add the cauliflower and the other ingredients toss bring to a simmer and cook over medium heat for 20 minutes more.

3. Blend the soup using an immersion blender, divide it into bowls and serve.

Nutrition:

Calories: 124

Total fat: 9g

Saturated fat: 8g

Sodium: 168mg

Carbs: 18g

Fiber: 8g

Protein: 6g

Rich Beans Soup

Preparation time: 10 minutes

Cooking time: 7 minutes

Servings: 4

Ingredients:
- 1 pound navy beans

- 1 yellow onion, chopped

- 4 garlic cloves, crushed

- 2 quarts veggie stock

- A pinch of sea salt

- Black pepper to the taste

- 2 potatoes, peeled and cubed

- 2 teaspoons dill, dried

    1 cup sun-dried tomatoes, chopped

-

- 1-pound carrots, sliced

- 4 tablespoons parsley, minced

Directions:

1. Put the stock in your slow cooker.

2. Add beans, onion, garlic, potatoes, tomatoes, carrots, dill, salt and pepper, stir, cover and cook on low for 7 hours.

3. Stir your soup, add parsley, divide into bowls and serve.

Nutrition:

Calories: 134

Total fat: 8g

Saturated fat: 5g

Sodium: 168mg

Carbs: 13g

Fiber: 8g

Protein: 6g

Mushroom Soup

Preparation time: 10 minutes

Cooking time: 7 minutes

Servings: 4

Ingredients:

- 1 onion (small, diced)

- 1 cup white button mushrooms (chopped)

- 1 cup Portobello mushrooms (stems removed, chopped)

- 2 cloves garlic (minced)

- 1/4 cup white wine

- 2 1/2 cups mushroom stock

- 2 tsp. salt and pepper

- 1 tsp. fresh thyme

- Cashew Cream:

- 1/2 cup raw cashews (soaked)

- 1/2 cup mushroom stock

Directions:

1. Add the onions and mushrooms to the pot, stirring every now and then, and set on "Sauté" mode for about 10 minutes (until the mushrooms have shrunk in size).

2. Add the garlic and sauté for 2 more minutes.

3. Add the wine and stir in until it evaporates and the smell of wine isn't as strong.

4. Add the salt, pepper, thyme, and mushroom stock, and stir. Cancel the sauté mode.

5. Put the lid on and put it on manual, setting the time to 5 minutes.

6. Add cashews and water into a blender, and blend until smooth. Release the pressure from the pot, remove the lid, and transfer to the blender and blend until smooth.

Nutrition:

Calories: 134

Total fat: 9g

Saturated fat: 5g

Sodium: 118mg

Carbs: 16g

Fiber: 8g

Protein: 6g

Cheesy Crackers

Preparation Time: 10 Minutes

Cooking Time: 20 Minutes

Servings: 3

Ingredients:

- 1 ¾ cup almond meal

- 3 tablespoons nutritional yeast

- ½ teaspoon of sea salt

- 2 tablespoons lemon juice

- 1 tablespoon melted coconut oil

- 1 tablespoon ground flaxseed

- 2 ½ tablespoons water

Directions:

1. Switch on the oven, then set it to 350 degrees F and let it preheat.

2. Meanwhile, take a medium bowl, place flaxseed in it, stir in water, and then let the mixture rest for 5 minutes until thickened.
3. Place almond meal in a medium bowl, add salt and yeast and then stir until mixed.
4. Add lemon juice and oil into the flaxseed mixture and then whisk until mixed.

5. Pour the flaxseed mixture into the almond meal mixture and then stir until dough comes together.

6. Place a piece of a wax paper on a clean working space, place the dough on it, cover with another piece of wax paper, and then roll dough into a 1/8-inch-thick crust.
7. Cut the dough into a square shape, sprinkle salt over the top and then bake for 15 to 20 minutes until done.
8. Serve straight away.

Nutrition:

Calories: 30 Cal;

Fat: 1 g;

Protein: 1 g;

Carbs: 5 g;

Fiber: 0 g

Tomato Soup

Preparation Time: 10 Minutes

Cooking Time: 10 Minutes

Servings: 2

Ingredients:

- 56 ounces stewed tomatoes

- ¼ teaspoon salt
- ¼ teaspoon ground black pepper
- 1 medium red bell pepper, cored, diced
- ¼ teaspoon dried thyme
- 6 leaves of basil, chopped
- ¼ teaspoon dried oregano
- 1 teaspoon olive oil

Directions:

1. Take a medium pot, place it over medium heat, add oil, and when hot, add bell pepper and then cook for 4 minutes.

2. Add remaining ingredients into the pot, stir until mixed, switch heat to medium-high heat, and bring the mixture to simmer.
3. Remove pot from the heat and then puree the soup until smooth.

4. Taste to adjust seasoning, ladle soup into bowls and then serve.

Nutrition:

Calories: 170 Cal;

Fat: 1.1 g;

Protein: 3.5 g;

Carbs: 36 g;

Fiber: 2.6 g

Meatballs Platter

Preparation Time: 10 Minutes

Cooking Time: 15 Minutes

Servings: 4

Ingredients:

- 1-pound beef meat, ground

- ¼ cup panko breadcrumbs

- A pinch of salt and black pepper

- 3 tablespoons red onion, grated

- ¼ cup parsley, chopped

- 2 garlic cloves, minced

- 2 tablespoons lemon juice

- Zest of 1 lemon, grated

- 1 egg

- ½ teaspoon cumin, ground

- ½ teaspoon coriander, ground

- ¼ teaspoon cinnamon powder

- 2 ounces feta cheese, crumbled

- Cooking spray

Directions:

1. In a bowl, blend the beef with the breadcrumbs, salt, pepper and the rest of the ingredients except the cooking spray, stir well and shape medium balls out of this mix.

2. Arrange the meatballs on a baking sheet lined with parchment paper, grease them with cooking spray and bake at 450 degrees F for 15 minutes.
3. Position the meatballs on a platter and serve as a snack.

Nutrition:

Calories: 300,

Fat: 15.4,

Fiber: 6.4,

Carbs: 22.4,

Protein: 35

Quick Zucchini Bowl

Preparation Time: 10 Minutes

Cooking Time: 10 Minutes

Servings: 4

Ingredients:

- ½ pound of pasta

- 2 tablespoons of olive oil

- 6 crushed garlic cloves

- 1 teaspoon of red chili

- 2 finely sliced spring onions

- 3 teaspoons of chopped rosemary

- 1 large zucchini cut up in half, lengthways and sliced

- 5 large portabella mushrooms

- 1 can of tomatoes

- 4 tablespoons of Parmesan cheese

- Fresh ground black pepper

Directions:

1. Cook the pasta.

2. Take a large-sized frying pan and place over medium heat.

3. Add oil and allow the oil to heat up.
4. Add garlic, onion and chili and sauté for a few minutes until golden.
5. Add zucchini, rosemary and mushroom and sauté for a few minutes.
6. Increase the heat to medium-high and add tinned tomatoes to the sauce until thick.

7. Drain your boiled pasta and transfer to a serving platter.
8. Pour the tomato mix on top and mix using tongs.
9. Garnish with Parmesan cheese and freshly ground black pepper.
   10.   Enjoy!

Nutrition:

Calories: 361

Fat: 12g

Carbohydrates: 47g

Protein: 14g

Healthy Basil Platter

Preparation Time: 25 Minutes

Cooking Time: 15 Minutes

Servings: 4

Ingredients:

- 2 pieces of red pepper seeded and cut up into chunks

- 2 pieces of red onion cut up into wedges

- 2 mild red chilies, diced and seeded

- 3 coarsely chopped garlic cloves

- 1 teaspoon of golden caster sugar

- 2 tablespoons of olive oil (plus additional for serving)

- 2 pounds of small ripe tomatoes quartered up

- 12 ounces of dried pasta

- Just a handful of basil leaves

- 2 tablespoons of grated Parmesan

Directions:

1. Pre-heat the oven to 392 degrees Fahrenheit.

2. Take a large-sized roasting tin and scatter pepper, red onion, garlic and chilies.

3. Sprinkle sugar on top.
4. Drizzle olive oil then season with pepper and salt.
5. Roast the veggies in your oven for 15 minutes.
6. Take a large-sized pan and cook the pasta in boiling, salted water until Al Dente.

7. Drain them.
8. Remove the veggies from the oven and tip in the pasta into the veggies.
9. Toss well and tear basil leaves on top.
   10.   Sprinkle Parmesan and enjoy!

Nutrition:

Calories: 452

Fat: 8g

Carbohydrates: 88g

Protein: 14g

Spiced Vegetable Couscous
Preparation Time: 10 minutes

Cooking Time: 20 minutes

Servings: 2

Ingredients

- Cauliflower – 1 head, cut into 1 –inch florets

- Extra-virgin olive oil – 6 tbsp. plus extra for serving

- Salt and pepper

- Couscous – 1 ½ cups

- Zucchini – 1, cut into ½ inch pieces

- Red bell pepper – 1, stemmed, seeded, and cut into ½ inch pieces

- Garlic – 4 cloves, minced

- Ras el hanout – 2 tsp.

- Grated lemon zest -1 tsp. plus lemon wedges for serving

- Chicken broth – 1 ¾ cups

- Minced fresh marjoram – 1 tbsp.

Directions

1. In a skillet, heat 2 tbsp. oil over medium heat.

2. Add cauliflowers, ¾ tsp. salt, and ½ tsp. pepper. Mix.
3. Cover and cook for 5 minutes, or until the florets start to brown and the edges are just translucent.
4. Remove the lid and cook, stirring for 10 minutes, or until the florets turn golden brown. Transfer to a bowl and clean the skillet.
5. Heat 2 tbsp. oil in the skillet.
6. Add the couscous. Cook and stir for 3 to 5 minutes, or until grains are just beginning to brown. Transfer to a bowl and clean the skillet.
7. Heat the remaining 3 tbsp. oil in the skillet and add bell pepper, zucchini, and ½ tsp. salt. Cook for 6 to 8 minutes, or until tender.
8. Stir in lemon zest, ras el hanout, and garlic. Cook until fragrant (about 30 seconds).
9. Stir in the broth and bring to a simmer.
10. Stir in the couscous. Cover, remove from the heat, and set aside until tender (about 7 minutes).
11. Add marjoram and cauliflower; then gently fluff with a fork to combine.
12. Drizzle with extra oil and season with salt and pepper.
13. Serve with lemon wedges.

Nutrition

Calories: 787

Fat: 18.3g

Carb: 129.6g

Protein: 24.5g

Pasta e Fagioli with Orange and Fennel

Preparation Time: 10 minutes

Cooking Time: 30 minutes

Servings: 5

Ingredients

- Extra-virgin olive oil – 1 tbsp. plus extra for serving

- Pancetta – 2 ounces, chopped fine

- Onion – 1, chopped fine

- Fennel – 1 bulb, stalks discarded, bulb halved, cored, and chopped fine

- Celery – 1 rib, minced
-
- Garlic – 2 cloves, minced
- Anchovy fillets – 3, rinsed and minced

- Minced fresh oregano – 1 tbsp.

- Grated orange zest – 2 tsp.

- Fennel seeds – ½ tsp.

- Red pepper flakes – ¼ tsp.

- Diced tomatoes – 1 (28-ounce) can

- Parmesan cheese – 1 rind, plus more for serving

  Cannellini beans – 1 (7-ounce) cans, rinsed

-

- Chicken broth – 2 ½ cups

- Water – 2 ½ cups

- Salt and pepper

- Orzo – 1 cup

- Minced fresh parsley – ¼ cup

Directions

1. Heat oil in a Dutch oven over medium heat. Add pancetta.

2. Stir-fry for 3 to 5 minutes or until beginning to brown.
3. Stir in celery, fennel, and onion and stir-fry until softened (about 5 to 7 minutes).
4. Stir in pepper flakes, fennel seeds, orange zest, oregano, anchovies, and garlic. Cook for 1 minute.

5. Stir in tomatoes and their juice. Stir in Parmesan rind and beans.
6. Bring to a simmer and cook for 10 minutes.
7. Stir in water, broth, and 1 tsp. salt.
8. Increase heat to high and bring to a boil.
9. Stir in pasta and cook for 10 minutes, or until al dente.
10. Remove from heat and discard parmesan rind.
11. Stir in parsley and season with salt and pepper to taste.
12. Drizzle with olive oil and sprinkle with grated Parmesan.
13. Serve.

Nutrition

Calories: 502

Fat: 8.8g

Carb: 72.2g

Protein: 34.9g

Cannellini Bean Soup with Kale

Preparation time: 10 minutes

Cooking Time: 25 minutes

Servings: 5

Ingredients:

- 1 tablespoon olive oil
- 1/2 teaspoon ginger, minced
- 1/2 teaspoon cumin seeds
- 1 red onion, chopped
  1 carrot, trimmed and chopped
- 1 parsnip, trimmed and chopped
- 2 garlic cloves, minced
- 5 cups vegetable broth
- 12 ounces Cannellini beans, drained
- 2 cups kale, torn into pieces
- Sea salt and ground black pepper, to taste

Directions:

1. In a heavy-bottomed pot, heat the olive over medium-high heat. Now, sauté the ginger and cumin for 1 minute or so.
2. Now, add in the onion, carrot and parsnip; continue sautéing an additional 3 minutes or until the vegetables are just tender.
3. Add in the garlic and continue to sauté for 1 minute or until aromatic.
4. Then, pour in the vegetable broth and bring to a boil. Immediately reduce the heat to a simmer and let it cook for 10 minutes.
5. Fold in the Cannellini beans and kale; continue to simmer until the kale wilts and everything is

thoroughly heated. Season with salt and pepper to taste.

6. Ladle into individual bowls and serve hot. Bon appétit!

Nutrition: Calories: 188; Fat: 4.7g; Carbs: 24.5g; Protein: 11.1g

Hearty Cream of Mushroom Soup

Preparation time: 10 minutes

Cooking Time: 15 minutes

Servings: 5

Ingredients:

- 2 tablespoons soy butter
- 1 large shallot, chopped
- 20 ounces Cremini mushrooms, sliced
- 2 cloves garlic, minced
- 4 tablespoons flaxseed meal
- 5 cups vegetable broth
- 1 1/3 cups full-fat coconut milk
- 1 bay leaf
- Sea salt and ground black pepper, to taste

Directions:

1. In a stockpot, melt the vegan butter over medium-high heat. Once hot, cook the shallot for about 3 minutes until tender and fragrant.
2. Add in the mushrooms and garlic and continue cooking until the mushrooms have softened. Add in the flaxseed meal and continue to cook for 1 minute or so.
3. Add in the remaining ingredients. Let it simmer, covered and continue to cook for 5 to 6 minutes more until your soup has thickened slightly.
4. Bon appétit!

Nutrition: Calories: 308; Fat: 25.5g; Carbs: 11.8g; Protein: 11.6g

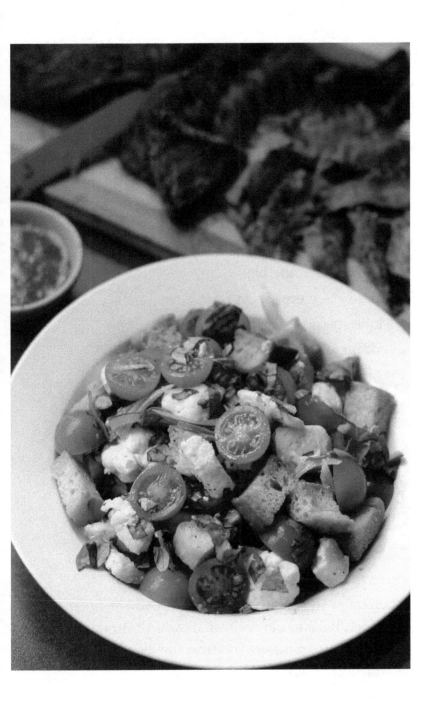

Authentic Italian Panzanella Salad

Preparation time: 10 minutes

Cooking Time: 35 minutes

Servings: 3

Ingredients:

- 3 cups artisan bread, broken into 1-inch cubes 3/4-pound asparagus, trimmed and cut into bite-sized pieces 4 tablespoons extra-virgin olive oil
- 1 red onion, chopped
- 2 tablespoons fresh lime juice
- 1 teaspoon deli mustard
- 2 medium heirloom tomatoes, diced
- 2 cups arugula
- 2 cups baby spinach
- 2 Italian peppers, seeded and sliced
- Sea salt and ground black pepper, to taste

Directions:

1. Arrange the bread cubes on a parchment-lined baking sheet. Bake in the preheated oven at 310 degrees F for about 20 minutes, rotating the baking sheet twice during the baking time; reserve.
2. Turn the oven to 420 degrees F and toss the asparagus with 1 tablespoon of olive oil. Roast the asparagus for about 15 minutes or until crisp-tender.

3. Toss the remaining Ingredients in a salad bowl; top with the roasted asparagus and toasted bread.

4. Bon appétit!

Nutrition: Calories: 334; Fat: 20.4g; Carbs: 33.3g; Protein: 8.3g

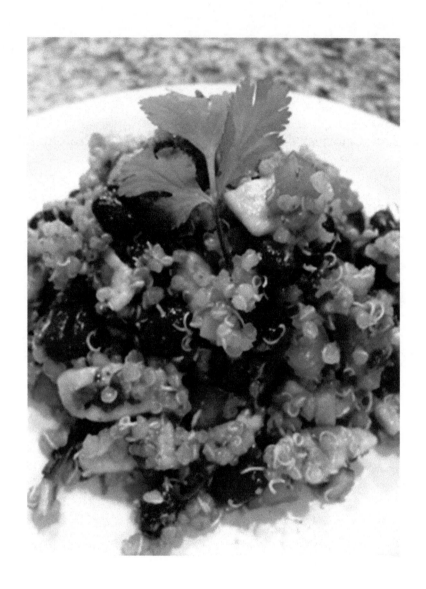

Quinoa and Black Bean Salad

Preparation time: 10 minutes
Cooking Time: 15 minutes + chilling time
Servings: 4
Ingredients:

- 2 cups water
- 1 cup quinoa, rinsed
- 16 ounces canned black beans, drained
- 2 Roma tomatoes, sliced
- 1 red onion, thinly sliced
- 1 cucumber, seeded and chopped
- 2 cloves garlic, pressed or minced
- 2 Italian peppers, seeded and sliced
- 2 tablespoons fresh parsley, chopped
  2 tablespoons fresh cilantro, chopped
- 1/4 cup olive oil
- 1 lemon, freshly squeezed
- 1 tablespoon apple cider vinegar
- 1/2 teaspoon dried dill weed
- 1/2 teaspoon dried oregano
- Sea salt and ground black pepper, to taste

Directions:

1. Place the water and quinoa in a saucepan and bring it to a rolling boil. Immediately turn the heat to a simmer.
2. Let it simmer for about 13 minutes until the quinoa has absorbed all of the water; fluff the quinoa with a fork and let it cool completely. Then, transfer the quinoa to a salad bowl.
3. Add the remaining Ingredients to the salad bowl and toss to combine well. Bon appétit!

Nutrition: Calories: 433; Fat: 17.3g; Carbs: 57g; Protein: 15.1g

Rich Bulgur Salad with Herbs

Preparation time: 10 minutes
Cooking Time: 20 minutes + chilling time
Servings: 4
Ingredients:

- 2 cups water
- 1 cup bulgur
- 12 ounces canned chickpeas, drained
- 1 Persian cucumber, thinly sliced
- 2 bell peppers, seeded and thinly sliced
- 1 jalapeno pepper, seeded and thinly sliced
- 2 Roma tomatoes, sliced
- 1 onion, thinly sliced
- 2 tablespoons fresh basil, chopped
- 2 tablespoons fresh parsley, chopped
- 2 tablespoons fresh mint, chopped
- 2 tablespoons fresh chives, chopped
- 4 tablespoons olive oil
- 1 tablespoon balsamic vinegar
- 1 tablespoon lemon juice
- 1 teaspoon fresh garlic, pressed
- Sea salt and freshly ground black pepper, to taste
- 2 tablespoons nutritional yeast
- 1/2 cup Kalamata olives, sliced

Directions:

1. In a saucepan, bring the water and bulgur to a boil. Immediately turn the heat to a simmer and let it cook for about 20 minutes or until the bulgur is tender and water is almost absorbed. Fluff with a fork and spread on a large tray to let cool.

2. Place the bulgur in a salad bowl followed by the chickpeas, cucumber, peppers, tomatoes, onion, basil, parsley, mint and chives.

3. In a small mixing dish, whisk the olive oil, balsamic vinegar, lemon juice, garlic, salt and black pepper. Dress the salad and toss to combine.

4. Sprinkle nutritional yeast over the top, garnish with olives and serve at room temperature. Bon appétit!

Nutrition: Calories: 408; Fat: 18.3g; Carbs: 51.8g; Protein: 13.1g

Classic Roasted Pepper Salad

Preparation time: 10 minutes

Cooking Time: 15 minutes + chilling time

Servings: 3

Ingredients:

- 6 bell peppers
- 3 tablespoons extra-virgin olive oil
- 3 teaspoons red wine vinegar
- 3 garlic cloves, finely chopped
- 2 tablespoons fresh parsley, chopped
- Sea salt and freshly cracked black pepper, to taste
- 1/2 teaspoon red pepper flakes
- 6 tablespoons pine nuts, roughly chopped

Directions:

1. Broil the peppers on a parchment-lined baking sheet for about 10 minutes, rotating the pan halfway through the cooking time, until they are charred on all sides.
2. Then, cover the peppers with a plastic wrap to steam. Discard the skin, seeds and cores.
3. Slice the peppers into strips and toss them with the remaining ingredients. Place in your refrigerator until ready to serve. Bon appétit!

Nutrition: Calories: 178; Fat: 14.4g; Carbs: 11.8g; Protein: 2.4g

Hearty Winter Quinoa Soup

Preparation time: 10 minutes
Cooking Time: 25 minutes
Servings: 4
Ingredients:

- 2 tablespoons olive oil
- 1 onion, chopped
- 2 carrots, peeled and chopped
- 1 parsnip, chopped
- 1 celery stalk, chopped
- 1 cup yellow squash, chopped
  4 garlic cloves, pressed or minced
- 4 cups roasted vegetable broth
- 2 medium tomatoes, crushed
- 1 cup quinoa
- Sea salt and ground black pepper, to taste
- 1 bay laurel
  2 cup Swiss chard, tough ribs removed and torn into
- pieces
- 2 tablespoons Italian parsley, chopped

Directions:

1.   In a heavy-bottomed pot, heat the olive over medium-high heat. Now, sauté the onion, carrot, parsnip, celery and yellow squash for about 3 minutes or until the vegetables are just tender.

2.   Add in the garlic and continue to sauté for 1 minute or until aromatic.

3.   Then, stir in the vegetable broth, tomatoes, quinoa, salt, pepper and bay laurel; bring to a boil. Immediately reduce the heat to a simmer and let it cook for 13 minutes.

4.   Fold in the Swiss chard; continue to simmer until the chard wilts.

5.   Ladle into individual bowls and serve garnished with the fresh parsley. Bon appétit!

Nutrition: Calories: 328; Fat: 11.1g; Carbs: 44.1g; Protein: 13.3g

Green Lentil Salad

Preparation time: 10 minutes

Cooking Time: 20 minutes + chilling time

Servings: 5

Ingredients:

- 1 ½ cups green lentils, rinsed
- 2 cups arugula
- 2 cups Romaine lettuce, torn into pieces
- 1 cup baby spinach
- 1/4 cup fresh basil, chopped
- 1/2 cup shallots, chopped
- 2 garlic cloves, finely chopped

  1/4 cup oil-packed sun-dried tomatoes, rinsed and chopped
- 5 tablespoons extra-
- virgin olive oil
- 3 tablespoons fresh lemon juice
- Sea salt and ground black pepper, to taste

Directions:

1.   In a large-sized saucepan, bring 4 ½ cups of the water and red lentils to a boil.

2.   Immediately turn the heat to a simmer and continue to cook your lentils for a further 15 to 17 minutes or until they've softened but not mushy. Drain and let it cool completely.

3.   Transfer the lentils to a salad bowl; toss the lentils with the remaining Ingredients until well combined.

4.   Serve chilled or at room temperature. Bon appétit!

Nutrition: Calories: 349; Fat: 15.1g; Carbs: 40.9g; Protein: 15.4g

Acorn Squash, Chickpea and Couscous Soup

Preparation time: 10 minutes

Cooking Time: 20 minutes

Servings: 4

Ingredients:

- 2 tablespoons olive oil
- 1 shallot, chopped
- 1 carrot, trimmed and chopped
- 2 cups acorn squash, chopped
- 1 stalk celery, chopped
- 1 teaspoon garlic, finely chopped
- 1 teaspoon dried rosemary, chopped
- 1 teaspoon dried thyme, chopped
- 2 cups cream of onion soup
- 2 cups water
- 1 cup dry couscous
- Sea salt and ground black pepper, to taste
- 1/2 teaspoon red pepper flakes
- 6 ounces canned chickpeas, drained
- 2 tablespoons fresh lemon juice

Directions:

1.   In a heavy-bottomed pot, heat the olive over medium-high heat. Now, sauté the shallot, carrot, acorn squash and celery for about 3 minutes or until the vegetables are just tender.

2.   Add in the garlic, rosemary and thyme and continue to sauté for 1 minute or until aromatic.

3.   Then, stir in the soup, water, couscous, salt, black pepper and red pepper flakes; bring to a boil.

Immediately reduce the heat to a simmer and let it cook for 12 minutes.

4.	Fold in the canned chickpeas; continue to simmer until heated through or about 5 minutes more.

5.	Ladle into individual bowls and drizzle with the lemon juice over the top. Bon appétit!

Nutrition: Calories: 378; Fat: 11g; Carbs: 60.1g; Protein: 10.9g

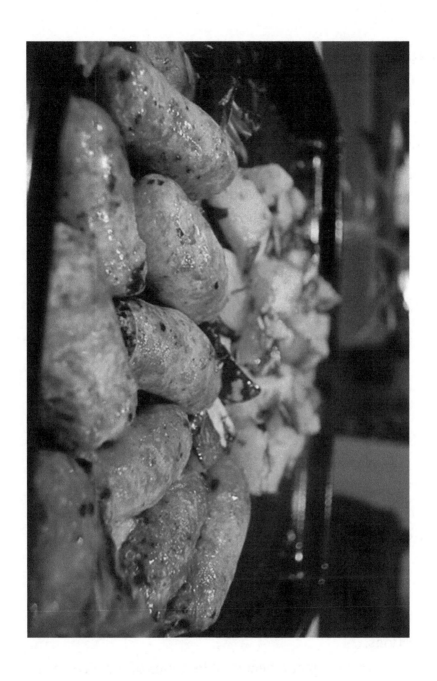

Cabbage Soup with Garlic Crostini

Preparation time: 10 minutes
Cooking Time: 1 hour
Servings: 4
Ingredients:

Soup:

- 2 tablespoons olive oil
- 1 medium leek, chopped
- 1 cup turnip, chopped
- 1 parsnip, chopped
- 1 carrot, chopped
- 2 cups cabbage, shredded
- 2 garlic cloves, finely chopped
- 4 cups vegetable broth
- 2 bay leaves
- Sea salt and ground black pepper, to taste
- 1/4 teaspoon cumin seeds
- 1/2 teaspoon mustard seeds
- 1 teaspoon dried basil
- 2 tomatoes, pureed

Crostini:

- 8 slices of baguette
- 2 heads garlic
- 4 tablespoons extra-virgin olive oil

Directions:

1.   In a soup pot, heat 2 tablespoons of the olive over medium-high heat. Now, sauté the leek, turnip, parsnip and carrot for about 4 minutes or until the vegetables are crisp-tender.

2.   Add in the garlic and cabbage and continue to sauté for 1 minute or until aromatic.

3.   Then, stir in the vegetable broth, bay leaves, salt, black pepper, cumin seeds, mustard seeds, dried basil and pureed tomatoes; bring to a boil. Immediately reduce the heat to a simmer and let it cook for about 20 minutes.

4.   Meanwhile, preheat your oven to 375 degrees F. Now, roast the garlic and baguette slices for about 15 minutes. Remove the crostini from the oven.

5.   Continue baking the garlic for 45 minutes more or until very tender. Allow the garlic to cool.

6.   Now, cut each head of the garlic using a sharp serrated knife in order to separate all the cloves.

7.   Squeeze the roasted garlic cloves out of their skins. Mash the garlic pulp with 4 tablespoons of the extra-virgin olive oil.

8.   Spread the roasted garlic mixture evenly on the tops of the crostini. Serve with the warm soup. Bon appétit!

Nutrition: Calories: 408; Fat: 23.1g; Carbs: 37.6g; Protein: 11.8g

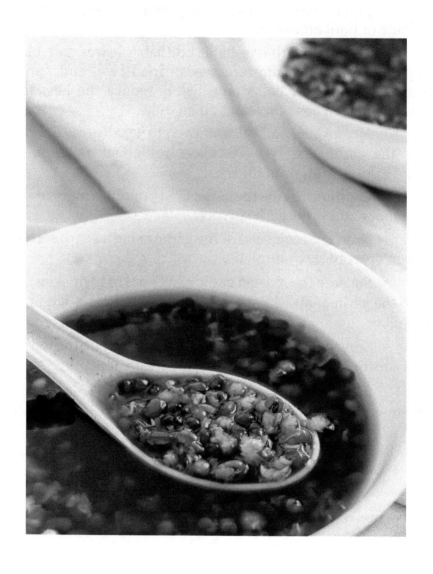

Chicken and Sausage Mix

Preparation Time: 10 Minutes
Cooking Time: 50 Minutes

Servings: 4

Ingredients:

- 2 zucchinis, cubed

- 1-pound Italian sausage, cubed

- 2 tablespoons olive oil

- 1 red bell pepper, chopped

- 1 red onion, sliced

- 2 tablespoons garlic, minced

- 2 chicken breasts, boneless, skinless and halved

- Salt and black pepper to the taste

- ½ cup chicken stock

- 1 tablespoon balsamic vinegar

Directions:

1. Heat up a pan with half of the oil over medium-high heat, add the sausages, brown for 3 minutes on each side and transfer to a bowl.

2. Heat up the pan again with the rest of the oil over medium-high heat, add the chicken and brown for 4 minutes on each side.
3. Return the sausage, add the rest of the ingredients as well, bring to a simmer, introduce in the oven and bake at 400 degrees F for 30 minutes.
4. Divide everything between plates and serve.

Nutrition:

Calories:293,

Fat:13.1,

Fiber:8.1,

Carbs:16.6,

Protein:26.1

Coriander and Coconut Chicken

Preparation Time: 10 Minutes

Cooking Time: 30 Minutes

Servings: 4

Ingredients:

- 2 pounds chicken thighs, skinless, boneless and cubed

- 2 tablespoons olive oil

- Salt and black pepper to the taste

- 3 tablespoons coconut flesh, shredded

- 1 and ½ teaspoons orange extract

- 1 tablespoon ginger, grated

- ¼ cup orange juice

- 2 tablespoons coriander, chopped

- 1 cup chicken stock

- ¼ teaspoon red pepper flakes

Directions:

1. Warmth up a pan through the oil over medium-high heat, add the chicken and brown for 4 minutes on each side.

2. Add salt, pepper and the rest of the ingredients, bring to a simmer and cook over medium heat for 20 minutes.
3. Divide the mix between plates and serve hot.

Nutrition:

Calories:297,

Fat:14.4,

Fiber:9.6,

Carbs:22,

Protein:25

Saffron Chicken Thighs and Green Beans

Preparation Time: 10 Minutes

Cooking Time: 25 Minutes

Servings: 4

Ingredients:

- 2 pounds chicken thighs, boneless and skinless

- 2 teaspoons saffron powder

- 1-pound green beans, trimmed and halved

- ½ cup Greek yogurt

- Salt and black pepper to the taste

- 1 tablespoon lime juice

- 1 tablespoon dill, chopped

Directions:

1. In a roasting pan, combine the chicken with the saffron, green beans and the rest of the ingredients, toss a bit, introduce in the oven and bake at 400 degrees F for 25 minutes.

2. Divide everything between plates and serve.

Nutrition:

Calories:274,

Fat:12.3,

Fiber:5.3,

Carbs:20.4,

Protein:14.3

Chicken and Olives Salsa

Preparation Time: 10 Minutes

Cooking Time: 25 Minutes

Servings: 4

Ingredients:

- 2 tablespoon avocado oil

- 4 chicken breast halves, skinless and boneless

- Salt and black pepper to the taste

- 1 tablespoon sweet paprika

- 1 red onion, chopped

- 1 tablespoon balsamic vinegar

- 2 tablespoons parsley, chopped

- 1 avocado, peeled, pitted and cubed

- 2 tablespoons black olives, pitted and chopped

Directions:
1. Heat up your grill over medium-high heat, add the chicken brushed with half of the oil and seasoned with paprika, salt and pepper, cook for 7 minutes on each side and divide between plates.

2. Meanwhile, in a bowl, mix the onion with the rest of the ingredients and the remaining oil, toss, add on top of the chicken and serve.

Nutrition:

Calories:289,

Fat:12.4,

Fiber:9.1,

Carbs:23.8,

Protein:14.3

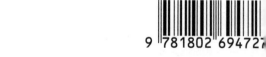